CW00841409

A Birth Path

stages & states of consciousness

~

B - A - Θ - Δ

~

by

HAZEL TREE

This book is a work of fiction and any resemblance to actual
persons, events or locales is entirely coincidental

Copyright 2016 ©Hazel Tree
ISBN: 978-1534716841
All rights reserved

The author asserts their moral right under the Copyright,
Designs and Patents Act, 1988, to be identified as the author of this work

All right reserved. No part of this publication may be reproduced,
copied, stored in a retrieval system or transmitted, in any form or by any
means, without the prior written consent of the copyright holder.

DEDICATION

This book is dedicated to the energy of birth, that mysterious power
that comes over birthing women and takes them on a journey
from the everyday to the mountain top.
Whether or not this is or will be our birthing experience
that energy is there, it dwells in all things.
It is in each of us.
It is us.

$$\tilde{}$$
$$\beta - \alpha - \theta - \Delta$$

$$\sim$$

CONTENTS

INTRODUCTION

B - A - $\tilde{\Theta}$ - Δ

~

7

The belief in a woman's ability to give birth unassisted is at the heart of this manual. Women have been doing so for generations upon generations, since the beginning of the human race in fact. And we have managed very well. Our existence is evidence to this. The natural process is to be trusted and allowed to unfold unless there are clear signs that mother and / or baby need help. Then medical interventions can be appreciated to be the wonderful life saving tools that they are. Once we understand what is normal then we can quickly detect the abnormal. This is done by studying the pattern, or path that birth normally follows.

The interesting challenge in writing a guidebook to the different states of labour is that each person's perception and experience is different. You may pass through some of these stages in a blur and not notice them happen and in others you may spend a long time getting to know that place very well. You may have all the symptoms, or few. There is a wide spectrum of normal; remember this is your body and no-one in the world knows it as well as you. For this reason, the next section is called *a* path to birth, not *the* path to birth because there are many, many paths. It is an archetypal journey in the sense that it is an original pattern; every birth follows this pattern but is not a true copy in that no two births are exactly the same. There are many factors that influence each woman and baby's individual path to birth. I hope that by understanding the archetypal journey you will understand your own some more as you follow in the footsteps of countless mothers before you.

In this book we will be following a possible path of normal labour and birth; that is one without any complications (as one could argue that *normal* could mean many things in our current medical climate). It is a sad fact of modern society that few women have had an opportunity to witness the birth process first hand until it happens to them. Then they are *in* the experience, which is very different.

Labour follows a common path known as the ***three stages of labour***. However please be aware this is not a definitive guide to how your labour will be; it is not something to aspire to, aim for, or judge your own labour by. Your labour will be as singular and unique as you are because it is shaped by your unique physiology, physical health, ancestral line, emotional state, mental state, home life, financial situation, birth environment, spiritual self, relationships and birth team. Even though birth is an involuntary biological process the link between body and mind is incredibly powerful. So powerful in fact that the mind and emotional state can affect the unfolding of labour, either consciously or unconsciously.

This manual is not a complete guide to labour and birth. It is intended to be used as part of a comprehensive preparation for birth and parenthood including self-knowledge and self-awareness practices. It is through direct experience that knowledge of one's own body signals and ability becomes clear. This preparation comes through experience and understanding of one's individual needs as well as self-defensive mechanisms in the face of stress, fear and pain. This is beyond right doing and wrong doing. When you understand your own ability together with an awareness of your choices you are on the path to having an authentic birth.

In this book we focus on of the stages and also *the states* of labour. I have attempted to explain what is happening internally and externally in the three main people involved in labour and birth: the mother, the baby and the father. Some of these explanations are physiological and some are written using creative license to convey how emotions, mind, body and spirit are linked in an inseparable way. Traditionally birth has been explained in medical terms of what was happening to the mother, the stages of labour marked by cervical dilation and so on. But there are many things going on during labour, on different levels of consciousness. In fact, one could say that labour cannot be defined in stages at all, but rather states, because labour essentially is about entering **altered states of consciousness.** The ordinary world is left behind as the path to birth is travelled, to return with a child.

For simplicity the birth partner is referred to as the *father* throughout. I understand the birth partner may be a female partner or perhaps a friend or relative supporting the mother during labour. In the same vein of understanding the baby is referred to as *she* throughout for consistency, although I understand that a baby can also be a boy! This section is written in the third person for accessibility.

By writing this manual I hope to explain in easy to understand steps how the path to birth is travelled. Take this to be a guidebook if you will; a description of a land far away that one day you, or someone you know, will visit and I hope understand for the incredible place that it is. I aim to set you up for success, to understand the different stages labour will pass through and what is happening in each one. Ultimately I wish you the confidence in yourself to trust your body to navigate the path to birth.

Blessings to you on your journey.

Hazel Tree

THE STAGES & STATES OF LABOUR

$$B - A - \overset{\sim}{\Theta} - \Delta$$
$\sim$

The Three Stages of Labour

There are traditionally three stages of labour used to refer to the physical changes that happen between the mother and baby during labour and birth.

In the **first** stage of labour the cervix softens from being as hard as the end of your nose, to as soft as your lips. Then contractions of the uterus, as well as the pressure of the descending baby, cause the cervix to open to around 10cm dilation.

During the **second** stage of labour the baby moves out of the uterus to travel down the birth canal and enter the pelvis. She then rotates and her presenting part becomes visible, which is normally the top of her head but can be feet, bottom, or face. She rotates again and is born.

In the **third** stage of labour contractions of the uterus and a change in hormones separate the placenta from the uterine wall. It then follows the path of the baby and is born.

The nine stages of labour as used in the *Birth Path*

First stage:
- Hearing the Call   - Pre-labour
- Beginning the Journey - Early labour
- Crossing the Threshold - Active labour
- Reaching the Summit   - Transition

Second stage:
- Space between worlds   - Rest & be Thankful
- The Road Home   - Pushing
- Welcome to the World - Crowning & Birth

Third stage:
- The Golden Hour   - Right after Birth
- Integration   - The Placenta Arrives

The Four States of Consciousness

Beta – Alpha – Theta – Delta

β - α - θ - Δ

The term *states* refers to the four levels of consciousness distinguishable by the frequency of the brainwave, measurable in Hertz.

It is often heard said that you cannot birth from your mind, and this is taken to mean that natural birth is more challenging when your mind is still functioning in the normal state of Beta, rather than the primal instinctive state of Theta. Beta is our regular waking consciousness, alert and active. There are three other states after Beta, namely: Alpha, Theta and Delta. During our daily life we move through all these states quite naturally although perhaps the shift we are most aware of is the move from waking to sleeping.

When we are aware of our surroundings, our place in the world and of the people around us we are in the state of Beta. Sensually this is the level of pre- or early arousal. In terms of waking or sleeping, while our brain is in Beta we are definitely awake. We are in our heads, thinking, analyzing, conscious of other people and the world around us. This is the realm of the neo-cortex, the intelligent sharp witty brain. It can be a challenge to birth while in the mental state of Beta because we are so aware of our surroundings.

If we were to use metaphor to understand these different states of being, in Beta we are standing at the ocean shore.

When the frequency of brain waves slow we move into what is known as Alpha state, a place of light relaxation, meditation and day-dreaming. This is a gateway state between the highly active and alert Beta and the sleeping Theta, it is the place you travel through as you lie down to sleep and mentally relax.

Sensually it is the place of high arousal and sexual intimacy where the rest of the world seems to melt away into the background. It could be said that this is the home of the intuitive voice, the lucid presence and awareness of knowing what is within. In this place we are more in touch with our bodies, our needs and wishes. Giving birth while in the state of Alpha can mean we are more in touch with ourselves and our baby, intuitively knowing what position to be in. It is a state of relaxation and surrender. There is still an awareness of the outer world and what is happening around but it is no longer of so much importance, it is like looking at the world through a window. Sounds can be muted; people's opinions matter little. Although it is possible to be drawn out of this state by bright lights and lots of questioning or by perceived danger. Any amount of adrenalin will change the state of awareness bringing it back up to Beta in case action is required.

Metaphorically Alpha is where we are in the ocean and swimming with the waves. In birthing this is where you let go of the outer world and begin to find the inner rhythm and connection with the Energy of Birth within.

The seat of deep peace and total calm lies in the state of Theta. There is no thinking here as this is the primal brain, the feeling instinctive place that is even more relaxed than Alpha. The outer world has drifted away and consciousness is very much centred within. For those attending a woman in labour this is where they can possibly feel left out as the mother journeys on alone. But their presence is essential, they are protecting the space, holding a state of external calm that gives the mother the space she needs to feel deeply safe so she may go within.

This is the state of consciousness you experience each night as light sleep. It is deeply restful for your mind as it no longer has to take in new stimulus from your senses. This is the state surrender known as orgasm.

Metaphorically Theta is where you are now riding the waves of the ocean.

Delta is an exquisite state of consciousness. Each of us experiences it every night as deep sleep but to experience it while awake is a cosmic experience not easily forgotten. It is a complete dissolution of the self and oneness with the divine, also called bliss or ecstasy. It is the state of consciousness that has direct contact with the unconscious, the place that dreams come from, as well as the collective unconscious, our collective dreaming. It is multiple orgasm. It is deep sleep.

It is the dissolution of separation between you and the ocean, you become one with the wave.

A summary of the states of consciousness

Beta brainwaves: β
- Frequency of 14 - 28 cycles per second / 16 – 31 Hz
- The thinking / rational conscious mind
- Active and alert, conversational
- Early arousal
- Awake
- Standing at the ocean shore

Alpha brainwaves: α
- Frequency of 7 - 14 cycles per second / 8 – 15 Hz
- A day-dreaming state, Light relaxation, meditation
- Lucid, not thinking
- A bridge between Beta and Theta
- Erotic intimacy
- Swimming in the ocean with the waves

Theta: θ
- Frequency of 4 – 7 cycles per second / 4 – 7 Hz
- Very deep relaxation. No thinking, all feeling, primal brain
- Absolute perfect calm
- The subconscious mind
- Orgasmic
- Light sleep
- Riding the ocean waves

Delta: Δ
- Frequency of 0 - 4 cycles per second / 0.1 – 3 Hz
- Cosmic bliss and oneness with the divine
- Ecstasy
- Multiple orgasm
- Deep sleep
- Becoming one with the wave

The First Stage of Labour

Where the mother's cervix softens and opens to full dilation

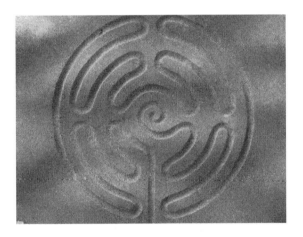

Hearing the call
Preparing for the journey
Crossing the threshold
Reaching the Summit

1 HEARING THE CALL

~ PRE-LABOUR

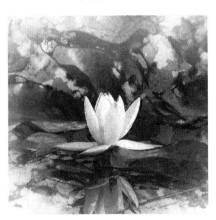

Mother
Beta – alpha consciousness

Mind awareness
Something is happening, she is sure of it, she has feelings that are different to before, there are new sensations and excitement bubbling like a stream has erupted in the middle of her tranquil garden. Her mind is buzzing and awake, beta brainwaves question and search for answers. Is this it? Am I in labour? She flits around the house like a dragonfly, folding some clothes here, cleaning a cupboard there. Her mind is only half on these tasks, the other half tingles with the truth dawning that this is it. She is going to have a baby! She might be telling everyone, waking her partner up in the middle of the night and phoning her mum. Or she might be quietly smiling to her herself, hugging the secret close during these last private moments alone. Time can go ever so slow when one is waiting for something to arrive sometimes. She decides to go back to sleep, or at least to lie down and rest, to slip back into alpha. She dreams vivid dreams.

Body awareness
There are some physical signs that labour is imminent. Maybe the plug of mucus that has acted as a barrier between uterine membranes and vagina has come away in a 'show'; brown, pink with a little blood. Maybe the membranes have released with a gush of sweet smelling clear liquid. Maybe contractions or surges have woken mother up in the middle of the night with a change from the Braxton-hicks' contractions she was getting to a stronger ache with pain sensations. The surges are irregular, coming many minutes or even hours apart but are important shifting and lifting contractions. These work together with the baby to shift her and lift her into the perfect position to enter the birth canal. Getting the right position can mean a smoother journey later. Mother helps by moving around, listening to her body's cues, keeping her knees lower than her hips and leaning forward to give baby as much room as possible to turn. In bed she uses pillows between her knees.

There are other invisible changes taking place inside mother's body during pre-labour. A high level of the hormone prostaglandin causes the cervix to change shape, soften and thin from a long, hard 'nose' to soft, thin 'lips.' This pre-labour thinning is essential before dilation can begin. Increased prostaglandins can also trigger extra bowel movements as well at this time. She eats well, hungry and with thirst.

This stage may take many hours, or days, as long as the two bodies need to prepare themselves for the journey that is to come.

She is approaching the ocean.

Baby

Mind awareness
For the last nine months or so baby has grown inside a warm bubble filled with sweet salty liquid. Her world has been filled with sounds of her mother's heartbeat and gurgling digestive system. She has somersaulted, twisted and turned while listening to the voices of people living their lives outside. Baby has felt the emotions of her mother via the bloodstream: happiness comes as oxytocin, stress and fear as adrenalin.

There is no coldness in this place, no hunger, no aloneness. She is always held tight, surrounded by the gently stretchy skin of her mother.

She seems to know exactly what she wants.

Body awareness
Her hands open and close, she plays with her umbilical cord and sucks her thumb. Being the heaviest part of her body, baby's back is where her centre of gravity lies. Her instinctive nature knows that the best position for her to approach the birth canal is with the left hand side of her head facing forward (left occiput anterior – LOA). She knows this fact to be so true that she will continue shifting and lifting until she is satisfied that she is approaching the cervix the right way. If the membranes have released and the amniotic fluids have gone then baby will now be directly touching skin for the first time in her life.

Father

Mind awareness

He knows that his partner is pregnant but he is still a little surprised when woken in the middle of the night and told it's happening. What, now? He leaps up and rushes around. Then slowly relaxes when he remembers that this is pre-labour which means the baby is letting them know she's getting ready. But there's time enough already. The nervous excitement ebbs and is replaced by a sense of calm. Mother and father find themselves alone to say goodbye to each other as they were, the stage of life when it was just the two of them is ending. They find they want to honour it in their own way.

They might feel called to spend the time connecting sensually and sharing sexual intimacy. This could also be a space for quiet reflection and meditation, a mental gathering together before the journey begins.

As time passes the family pull into themselves, drawing in those needed around them during this time. Depending on habits and preferences they will let their caregivers, friends and family know that birth is imminent. The final arrangements are made. There could be a nesting urge to clean and tidy the home, that final fling to prepare the space for this new person who will soon be arriving into the middle of everything. Father puts up that shelf, or mends that door, or puts away the tools he's been meaning to do. There may be excitement or nervous anticipation of what is to come.

Body awareness

The father is affected by and can affect the hormones in the mother. Relaxation and warm loving feelings produce oxytocin which aids the labour process, His understanding of the link between mind and body in this way help him to prepare the environment so that it is conducive for oxytocin flow to ease out of beta thinking into alpha feeling state consciousness.

2 BEGINNING THE JOURNEY

~ EARLY LABOUR

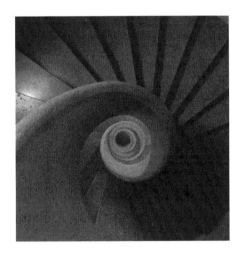

Mother
Beta – alpha level of consciousness.

Mind awareness:
The waves of contractions begin and mother knows the journey has begun. Her mind is working on Beta wavelength – the thinking mind is switched on and conscious. In between surges she will be able to continue a conversation; she shares explanations of her physical sensations with the people around her. Simple tasks like cooking, tidying, and taking a walk work to occupy her mind before the labour takes her away on its journey. It can be tempting after waiting so many months for this journey to begin to surrender every bit of attention to the physical sensations. The danger here is mind exhaustion as she worries about the growing intensity of the surges. The journey may yet be long, how will she cope if this is still early labour? She holds the awareness lightly in her mind, not giving it her full attention yet. The alpha state calls her; she surrenders, trusting the energy of birth. She knows that her body will release endorphins to counter the pain. She fills the bath with hot water and slips in, eyes gently close. Welcoming the growing energy that will enable her to birth her baby.

At the shore she stands and contemplates the ocean before her.

Body awareness/ physical signs:
The rush of adrenalin that comes with the awareness that 'this is it' can cause a lot of physical activity rushing around getting things ready. Mother remembers that this stage can last a long time and that the hormone oxytocin (which is a 'shy' hormone) must be nurtured through quiet and relaxation. Adrenalin can inhibit the progression of labour. She uses her breath to focus and calm her body. The hormone relaxin aids the connective tissues in the cervix to soften as it prepares to open, the whole body is at its most flexible and naturally capable of relaxing. The increasing levels of endorphins stimulate the release of prolactin which in turn stimulates breastfeeding. Her body is preparing to nurse her newborn.

31

Surges can be anything from 5 to 20 minutes apart and between 10 to 45 seconds long. There will be varying degrees of sensations and pain experienced. It may be menstrual-like cramping, or increased discomfort or maybe a deep sense of relaxation and bliss as the sensations wash over her. The two reliable signs of labour progressing beyond pre-labour are noticeable contractions with a regular, consistent pattern.

The cervix swings forwards and dilates to about 4 or 5cm. At some stage either now or later, maybe not until the moment of birth, the membranes will release and there will be a gush of sweet smelling, clear amniotic fluid.

Baby

Mind awareness:
Baby has been able to hear since she was 25 weeks old; she knows the voices of her mother and father intimately. She has a range of emotions but her natural state is one of quiet meditative alertness. All her nine months of life she has lived in perfect bliss, with all her physical needs being instantly cared for. She has never known cold, or hunger or loneliness. Now things are beginning in a completely new way. Her mother has been anticipating a big event and now it is here. There are new feelings of excitement and sensations of tightening.

Body awareness:
Baby has reached the stage of her physical development where she is ready to be born. Her brain and hormonal system work seamlessly with her mother's body. Baby's hormonal system works to compensate fear by releasing endorphins and adrenalin if shocked or stressed. These changes can be detected through listening to her heart beat, as well as intuitively. Research has shown that labour is physically initiated by an enzyme from baby's lungs which cause more prostaglandins to be released into the mother's system, beginning the thinning and softening of the cervix before dilation as well as initiating contractions. It could also be said to be initiated by baby's will to be born or as a physical manifestation of the creative power of the universe. However it is perceived - birth is happening.

Father

Mind awareness:
Fears and anxieties may surface as suddenly everything becomes more real. Father connects with the birthing mother. He is close by, letting her talk if she needs to. His calm presence is communicated through word, attitude, body language and touch. He is prepared. He has his own support network and knows who to call if he needs to. The father understands that this is early labour and stays calm, conserving his energy. His attention also goes to preparing the environment, making it conducive to the energy of birth. He knows she needs to feel safe, warm and loved while she travels to collect the soul of their child and bring it though birth. He has educated himself and understands how birth works to be able to hold this protective space around her.

Body awareness:
There may be adrenalin knowing that labour is beginning but he knows how to relax his body. This is a wonderful time to be intimate with the mother of his child, they kiss, hug, massage her breasts and make love. Penetration is safe as long as the membranes have not released. All kinds of love-making increase oxytocin which assists in the natural flow of birthing hormones. They do what feels good.

3 CROSSING THE THRESHOLD

~ ACTIVE LABOUR

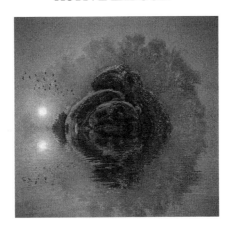

Mother
Alpha - theta

Mind awareness:
Mother has left behind the everyday world and walks on the path to birth. This takes up her awareness. Walking deep within she craves privacy, quiet and dim light more. She needs to trust that she is safe, loved and has all the privacy she needs. Light conversation has stopped, a sense of serious concentration descends. She looks to her birth partner, the father of her child to know that he is with her. They may speak without words, finding the rhythm of the dance and connect together with the presence of their baby. Their sensual intimacy is heightened, skin is sensitive to touch. The rest of the world seems to fade out of focus and into the background. Deep in the primal brain she loses inhibition and sheds her clothes without a thought.

Sometimes she drifts off alone, unaware of anyone else in the room, to be alone with these building sensations that are claiming her body. Eyes glaze over and close, she walks between worlds and seeks the soul of her child.

Breathing will be a welcome vehicle to focus the mind and in the present moment. The thing calling her is to find the rhythm of the dance: a way to ride the surges, to keep her courage and strength while relaxing and opening completely to surrender to the increasing powerful surges. She is directly experiencing the creative power of the universe. The intensity is incredible. There is no turning back only going onwards and upward.

She is climbing the mountain. She is swimming in the ocean with the waves.

Body awareness:
Contractions are closer together and more intense as cervical dilation continues. The surges may be 3 - 4 minutes apart and 40 – 60 seconds long.

Hormones continue to flood her body with a mixture of endorphins to control the pain sensations and prostaglandin to encourage effective contractions. During each contraction oxygen flow to the uterus stops; this lack of oxygen in the muscles is one source of pain sensations. In between surges there is a strong need to rest as this will increase blood flow to the uterus and she will find her own comfortable position, maybe kneeling or resting against her birth partner. Breathing will become a very important anchor in the present moment, for the mind and also to increase oxygenated blood flow. There will be thirst but probably not hunger.

Deeply in touch with the needs of her body she moves and uses sound to release tension in the pelvic floor. In her heightened state of theta she unconsciously understands the neurological connection between throat and vagina. She opens her throat with sound, which also opens her vagina. Stress hormones could restrict endorphins and oxytocin as well as constricting the muscles around the opening of the cervix, so she works to find ways to release any stress or tension over and over again.

Baby

Mind awareness:
The feelings and awareness that baby is experiencing during labour are unique to her. She may find pleasure in the rhythmic contractions that massage her body, or she may find their intensity frightening. She listens to her mother sounding and to the comforting voice of her father close by.

Body awareness:
The contractions continue to shift and lift baby during this stage of labour. Her body is still finding her way towards the best position to navigate the birth canal as the cervix dilates. In between the contractions she feels a flood of oxygenated blood fill her body. During contractions the blood flow slows and she uses glucose from her own body stores to give her energy. The uterus is tighter around her than it has ever been and her body folded up as small as it can be.

Father

Mind awareness:
The father understands where mother has gone, he knows her wishes and it is his job to protect the space. He holds the energy and is her guardian creating an environment conductive to birth, which is much like a love-making environment. He is finding new levels of intimacy with her as they swim in the ocean of labour together. She is glowing and he bathes in the light. Breath for breath he breathes with her, feeling the intensity of the experience build. Their kisses are passionate and rich.

When she drifts off alone he does not disturb her. He keeps her privacy, maintains the quiet and low lighting.

Body awareness:
The father's body is also experiencing a hormonal rush and is full of oxytocin and endorphins. Together they sway and dance. He strokes her arm while she rests between surges offering her a sip of something to drink.

4 REACHING THE SUMMIT

~ TRANSITION

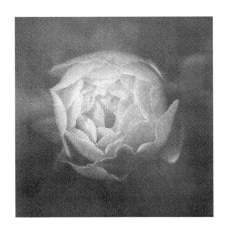

Mother
Alpha - theta - delta

Mind awareness:
This can be the most challenging part of her journey, the part where mother doubts herself, cries out in pain and says she can't go on. She loses her rhythm, nothing works anymore, she asks for drugs and makes lots of noise. The energy changes. Eyes may become wild open seeking for help to cross the threshold. She thinks of her own mother and their relationship.

She is the storm raging. She is the primal force of nature wild and untameable. She has reached the summit of the mountain and from here calls down the soul of her child to walk the path down to life. It can be empowering or vulnerable and confusing.

She fears she might be drowning under the waves.

Body awareness:
Her cervix is at 10cm dilation, this is as physically open as a woman can be. Contractions change, becoming longer and more intense. The emotionally charged atmosphere stimulates a release of adrenalin which boosts energy and stimulates the foetal ejection reflex that assists birth. She may shake to release tension or vomit, which causes the diaphragm to push against the top of the uterus aiding the process. The membranes may release if they haven't already.
This is the peak, the most intense sensations of pain are experienced now. The name transition is accurate because the uterus is transitioning from opening the cervix to pushing the baby down the birth canal. She may be in pain, but need not be suffering.

Baby

Mind awareness:
During pregnancy and labour mother and baby are as one. They share blood and its cocktail of hormones. When one feels calm so

43

does the other. Imagine then how it is for baby right now during transition when the energy is at its most intense and tension is high. And then the moment of surrender comes and the energy moves again.

Body awareness:
Each contraction pulls up the cervix which presses on baby's head. This stimulates her to wriggle and push against it as the cervix opens, it is like a jumper being pulled tightly around her head. There are not many nerves on the top of her head and she may still be protected by the cushion of amniotic fluid. Each contraction squeezes her body sending messages telling her body to prepare for life outside the womb.

Father

Mind awareness:
In this moment of changing winds the mind and heart can question itself. The father may feel tired and wonder how much longer this will last, he is concerned that mother no longer seems able to cope. But now is the time for him to stand strong, to breathe deep and hold his faith in her. The mother needs love and reassurance that she is doing well and surrounded by people she can trust. Father doesn't try to relax or calm her. She may actually need the freedom to shout and scream and release any fears and tension. If she is scared and lost the father will be there to remind her what an amazing job she is doing. She is travelling the path to birth and she is nearly there. He doesn't take anything she says personally, if there are angry words said he lets them go and moves on. The tides are turning.

Body awareness:
The father takes responsibility for his own welfare. Protecting his posture, especially if the mother is using him as support, he uses chairs or the wall to support himself. He keeps breathing and stays open and present to what is happening in the moment. This might not be what was planned, but he is ready for anything.

The Second Stage of Labour

Where the baby travels down the birth canal and is born

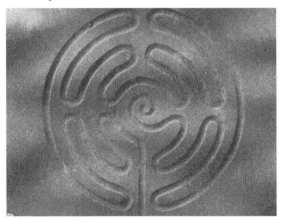

Space between worlds
Bringing spirit home
Welcoming

5 SPACE BETWEEN WORLDS

~ REST & BE THANKFUL

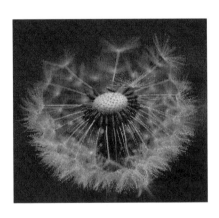

Mother
Alpha - theta - delta

Mind awareness:
This is the calm after the storm. Mother has reached the highest point of the path, has touched heaven and now pauses to breathe in the magnificence of creation. She has done the hard work of opening and now an eternal moment is touched. The rest is welcomed and her mood changes as the skies clear. She is calmer.

She is in the eye of the storm.

Body awareness:
Contractions pause. Mother may rest here for 10 – 30 minutes, or the moment may pass by. Either way the change in energy is noticeable. The cervix is fully dilated. The uterus uses this time to shorten. Brain waves slow even more, she may reach the deepest place of Delta waves, the oneness of ecstatic bliss and complete unity.

Baby

Mind awareness:
Baby rests, maybe she sleeps a little now the walls of the uterus have slowed their massage. She knows the time of birth is near. She is perfectly lined up with the bones of her mother's pelvis.

Body awareness:
The baby's head has passed out of the uterus and now lies in the birth canal. Only her body remains inside the loosely fitting uterus now the biggest bit of her body has passed through. The uterus uses this resting time to tighten around her again.

Father

Mind awareness:
The father is also resting in moments of bliss in this time between time. He feels relieved that transition has passed and knows that this is the space to gather energy for the next stage.

Body awareness:
Now is the time for the father to also rest and be thankful. Let the body do what it needs to get ready before the next stage. He eats and marvels at how good it tastes.

6 THE ROAD HOME

~ BEARING DOWN

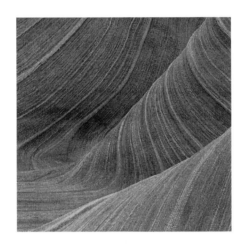

Mother
Alpha - theta - delta

Mind awareness:
A corner has been turned and the journey home lies ahead. Mother is filled with a new sense of purpose: bringing her baby home. All her energy is inward, working intensely with effective contractions that bear baby down the birth canal. She straddles the worlds of consciousness and subconsciousness.

With all of her senses heightened, she can hear things whispered, detect tones and sub-meanings with vivid clarity. Everything that happens around and inside her is part of her awareness. She is the woman who knows. In private communication mother and baby work together to navigate the final twists of the birth passage. She is a maiden crossing the threshold to motherhood bringing deep wisdom that will stay with her for the rest of her days. She is a chrysalis transforming. She is alive, as well as a vehicle for new life, a channel for the birth energy. She is a birthing goddess resplendent in all her glory. Roaring like a lion as she bears down.

She is riding the wave.

Body awareness:
Contractions change from opening to bearing down. Their energy is powerful and intense. Adrenalin and endorphins are released into the bloodstream. Baby's head descends to the pelvic floor muscles towards the perineum.

The length of the birth canal is about the same as the cervix at full dilation -10cm. The pelvis has become more flexible with increased amounts of relaxin and the front joint of the pelvis opens up to allow baby to pass through. The birth canal engorges with blood and pushes the bladder forward and the rectum back to allow maximum space for the birth canal. The urge to push begins slowly with a grunt caught in the back of her throat. The movement down grows stronger the more baby's head descends. Her behaviour is guided by her instincts, the urge to push becomes all encompassing. She uses the force of gravity.

In time the sounds she makes change to become deep grunting and pushing sounds.

In between contractions she rests deeply.

Baby

Mind awareness:
The journey changes tempo now as baby leaves her uterine home and moves down the birth canal. The journey is slow and this gives her time to twist and turn navigating her way. She feels the pull of gravity in a different way as she is no longer floating in the womb waters.

Body awareness:
Being perfectly designed for birth baby's skull bones overlap and mould to fit the birth canal. The placenta behind her is still connected to the uterine wall and continues to give oxygen. The vaginal walls surround her face muffling the sounds of her mother roaring. Each contraction of uterus slowly pushes her down towards the circle of light her eyes can see waiting. The tightening of the birth canal massages her lungs loosening and preparing them for their imminent entry into the world of air. There is a lot of pressure. Baby's skin is colonised with maternal bacteria which helps her immune system to develop. She is tired.

Father

Mind awareness:
The father is swept up in the energy of the labour now, thoughts of the outside world put aside and the work of the birthing mother fills his heart and soul. He is renewed and awake, encouraging her, telling her how well she is doing after each contraction that brings them one step closer to meeting their baby for the first time. It is an emotional time with the reality coming closer, yet still being in a bubble of concentration surrounding the mother.

Body awareness:

He stays aware of his body, his arms tire and he gently changes position. He uses pillows under his knees and cushions behind his back to be comfortable while staying present to the mother's needs. He remembers the birth wishes plan, reminds the medical caregivers if need be. The receiving blanket is ready.

7 WELCOME TO THE WORLD

~ CROWNING & BIRTH

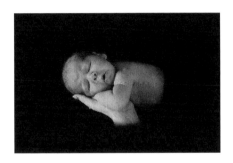

Mother
Alpha - theta - delta

Mind awareness:
There is little mind in this moment, the intense physical sensations of stretching take up full awareness. Mother knows the baby is there, she reaches down with a hand to feel the top of the head. She knows there is no one correct position in which to give birth to her baby, only the one that feels right in the moment. Her mind and body are so close, they are one. She acts without thinking, without analysis. She knows. She is ecstasy incarnated. She is the wave.

Body awareness:
Mother has found the position in which she wants to give birth. She kneels on one knee, her hands free to catch the baby. She knows her caregivers are close by if needed. Her pelvis is open; her coccyx has rolled back out of the way. The rate of descent and emergence into the world is controlled and careful. The vagina is stretched to its physical limit, the perineum burns like a ring of fire as her baby's head crowns and this time does not return inside. Adrenalin rushes through her bloodstream. Oxytocin flows. She cries out and arches her back rising slightly, the head emerges. A moment or an eternity later the rest of her baby is born. The mother has done it, this amazing incredible thing, she has given birth!

Baby

Mind awareness:
Baby is swaddled in the soft warm folds of her mother's body but cannot stay here for too long. She is ready to come out. The tightening is intense now until finally the tunnel opens and she emerges into a different world. She has finished her time in the watery womb and is a child of air now. She takes a breath, and smells the air for the first time.

Body awareness:

Baby has been completely germ free while she lived in the sterile womb. Antibodies have been transferring to her through the placenta for the last few weeks to prepare her for this moment as she passes through the vagina and past her mother's anus. Baby's body is colonized by billions of 'friendly' germs from her mother to begin the normal and natural colonisation of her digestive tract setting her up for a healthy life outside.

The perineum is tight and needs time to gently stretch to allow her head to pass. Baby emerges then retreats again and again stretching the perineum a little more each time. The top of her head has passed through the gate of life. The skin on the scalp stretches tight. There is a drop in temperature. The contractions push. The membranes will release if they haven't already. Her face emerges. Her whole head is outside, facing towards her mother's back. There is a pause between contractions. Baby turns her whole body 45 degrees to one side then one shoulder comes out, followed by the rest of her body. She is fully manifest on the earth.

Father

Mind awareness:
As mother stretches physically the father can also stretch emotionally. This path to birth has been long, he has travelled many miles and at this final stage there are more emotions than he ever knew possible. He feels things on a new level. The meaning of love has changed as he goes through the transition into a new realm where he is a creator of life, participating in the birth of his creation. The first glimpse of his child's head as it emerges out of the vagina fills him with emotion. He prepares to meet his child.

The awe of the power of birthing energy will stay with him always. He is forever changed as he enters fatherhood.

Body awareness:
He stays close to the mother, connected and encouraging her through the crowning stretch. As baby emerges he may be next to mother's head using eye contact to keep her focused or he may watch the baby emerge from her vagina. He is intensely present.

The Third Stage of Labour

Where the placenta is born

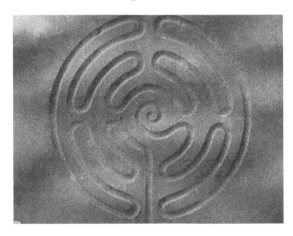

The Golden Hour
Integration

8 THE GOLDEN HOUR

~ BONDING AFTER BIRTH

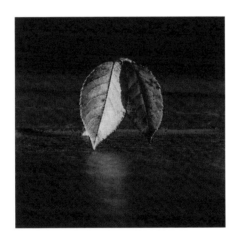

Mother
Beta - alpha - theta - delta

Mind awareness:
She has done it. She has travelled the path to other realms and now returns to put her feet on the Earth. Elation at her accomplishment, pride in herself fills her being. Then attention moves to this perfect being that has arrived. Mother's heart is full to overflowing with love for this child and for her partner.

Body awareness:
The oxytocin and endorphin love cocktail is pumping; she feels love like she has never known. The placenta is still attached to the wall of her womb.

Baby

Mind awareness:
Baby emerges from the birth canal and incredibly quickly adapts to life. Within minutes she has begun to breathe regularly. The world of smells is rich and diverse after the uterine environment. She opens her eyes and searches for the faces of the voices she knows so well. When she finds them she stares. She is deeply in love.

Body awareness:
Enormous changes are happening inside baby's body in the first few minutes' post-birth. She takes her first breath and begins the change from fetal circulation to neonatal circulation. She has travelled down the birth canal with only two thirds of her blood supply and fills up with the other third while her umbilical cord is still pulsing. The bluish tint to her skin turns pink as her blood levels rise. When she begins breathing prostaglandin from her lungs make the umbilical arteries contract and the flow of blood slowly decreases until the cord is white and floppy. Now it can be clamped and cut if desired.

Her skin is covered in patches of white, creamy vernix and perhaps patches of blood. Her skull needs some time to relax after being squeezed through the birth canal; this may take some days.

Father

Mind awareness:
The father moves in close to claim his family. These are emotions beyond words.

Body awareness:
The release of excess adrenalin may come through with tears or shaking. The flow of oxytocin increases and he falls in love even more deeply. He might need to remember to keep breathing.

9 INTEGRATION

~ THE ARRIVAL OF THE PLACENTA

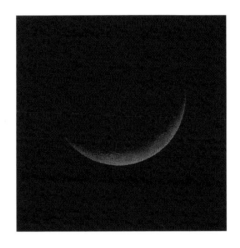

Mother

Beta - alpha

Mind awareness:
Mother is busy getting to know her baby with awe and reverence. She is still coming back down to earth. Together with the baby's father they explore this new person that has entered their lives.

Body awareness:
With her baby on her chest mother's skin temperature will adjust automatically to either warm baby if cold or cool her down if too warm. There are some contractions of the uterus and the placenta detaches from the uterine wall where it attached nine months ago. Blood gushes out from the site where the transfer from mother's blood and baby's blood has been taking place. The uterus continues to contract constricting the blood vessels and pushing the placenta down and out of the vagina. This contracting is aided by baby sucking on mother's breasts which releases oxytocin and encourages contractions. The birth of the placenta marks the end of the third stage of labour. The fourth trimester begins.

Baby

Mind awareness:
Baby is alert and highly aware in this period right after birth even though she is deeply tired from her journey to birth. Although she is small she is a whole person, bringing her own unique self into the world. In this moment her needs are paramount and she will use her communication skills to let those around her know what it is she needs to adjust to this new world. For her there is no difference between needs and wants, what she wants she needs and it will be quite some time before there is a separation.

She is falling in love with the new faces of her mother and father, their smells and the touch of their skin. She senses their emotions and is comforted by their presence and attention. The sound of her mother's heartbeat is instantly comforting as it has filled her world for the nine months of gestation.

Body awareness:
A flush of hormones encourages baby to stay awake and fall in love. There is so much space out here after the tightness of the womb! Her spine begins to uncurl, her arms stretch out for the first time, hands open to grasp onto whatever touches them. She can focus her vision at about 30cm, far enough to see the faces close to her. She easily feels the cold after the constant warmth inside, so enjoys the feeling of skin-to-skin on her mother's chest.

The smell of the breast calls to her instinctive nature and she bobs her head around rooting for the nipple. She has practised for this moment while in the womb, often sucking her hand. If the nipple is out of reach she will use her strong muscles to wriggle towards the breast. When she has the nipple in her mouth she begins to suck and is rewarded with feeling connected and close as well as tasting the warm thick sweetness of colostrum. The teaspoon amount is just enough for her tiny belly, it is full of goodness and satisfies her completely. It also contains antibodies and anti-infectious substances that enrich her gut flora, setting up her immune system. She falls asleep content. Her life is beginning.

Father

Mind awareness:
These early moments are hugely significant. The father touches and smells his baby for the first time. He realizes that she knows him already, turns to hear his voice and is comforted by his presence. Deep peace washes over him and he expands into the new identity of fatherhood.

Body awareness:
A new relationship begins when the father sees, smells and touches his daughter. The smell speaks to his body in a biological way beyond words. Their bonding is the beginning of the fourth trimester.

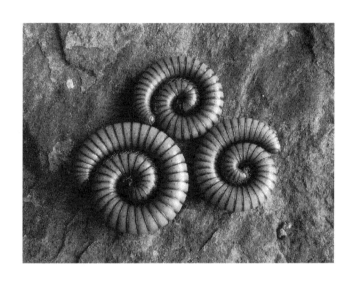

About the author

Hazel Tree is fascinated by the interplay between brain waves and the human experience, especially surrounding childbirth. She is a doula, childbirth educator and author of the novel 'A Doula's Journey.' She lives in Devon with her partner and son where she divides her time between working on their organic smallholding, being a birthworker and facilitating women's circles.

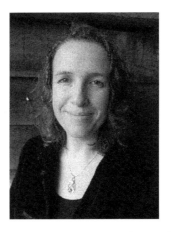

www.authenticbirth.co.uk

Bibliography

- Empowering Women by Andrea Robertson
- Pregnant Feelings by Rahima Baldwin & Terra Palmarini Richardson
- Ina May's Guide to Childbirth by Ina May Gaskin
- The Birth Partner by Penny Simkin
- Effective Birth Preparation by Maggie Howell
- Birth and beyond by Dr Yehudi Gordon
- Birthing from within by Pam England
- The Secret Life of the unborn Child by Dr Thomas Verny with John Kelly
- New Active Birth by Janet Balaskas
- The Transition to Parenthood by Jay Belsky and John Kelly
- Preparing for Birth and Parenthood by Gerlinde M. Wilberg
- The truth about illness, unhappiness and stress? by Barry & Winnie Durbant-Hollamby
- The Caesarean by Michel Odent

18511343R00046

Printed in Great Britain
by Amazon